Blood Pressure Monitoring Chart

Month _____

Date	Time	Systolic / Diastolic		Pulse
		/		
		/		
		/		
		/		
		/		
		/		
		/		
		/		
		/		
		/		
		/		
		/		
		/		
		/		

Blood Pressure Monitoring Chart

Month _____

Date	Time	Systolic	/	Diastolic	Pulse
			/		
			/		
			/		
			/		
			/		
			/		
			/		
			/		
			/		
			/		
			/		
			/		
			/		

Blood Pressure Monitoring Chart

Month _____

Date	Time	Systolic / Diastolic	Pulse
		/	
		/	
		/	
		/	
		/	
		/	
		/	
		/	
		/	
		/	
		/	
		/	
		/	
		/	

Blood Pressure Monitoring Chart

Month _____

Date	Time	Systolic / Diastolic		Pulse
			/	
			/	
			/	
			/	
			/	
			/	
			/	
			/	
			/	
			/	
			/	
			/	
			/	
			/	

Blood Pressure Monitoring Chart

Month _____

Date	Time	Systolic	/	Diastolic	Pulse
			/		
			/		
			/		
			/		
			/		
			/		
			/		
			/		
			/		
			/		
			/		
			/		
			/		
			/		

Blood Pressure Monitoring Chart

Month _____

Date	Time	Systolic / Diastolic		Pulse
			/	
			/	
			/	
			/	
			/	
			/	
			/	
			/	
			/	
			/	
			/	
			/	
			/	
			/	

Blood Pressure Monitoring Chart

Month _____

Date	Time	Systolic / Diastolic		Pulse

Blood Pressure Monitoring Chart

Month _____

Date	Time	Systolic / Diastolic	Pulse
		/	
		/	
		/	
		/	
		/	
		/	
		/	
		/	
		/	
		/	
		/	
		/	
		/	
		/	

Blood Pressure Monitoring Chart

Month _____

Date	Time	Systolic	/	Diastolic	Pulse
			/		
			/		
			/		
			/		
			/		
			/		
			/		
			/		
			/		
			/		
			/		
			/		
			/		
			/		

Blood Pressure Monitoring Chart

Month _____

Date	Time	Systolic / Diastolic		Pulse

Blood Pressure Monitoring Chart

Month _____

Date	Time	Systolic / Diastolic		Pulse

Blood Pressure Monitoring Chart

Month _____

Date	Time	Systolic / Diastolic		Pulse
		/		
		/		
		/		
		/		
		/		
		/		
		/		
		/		
		/		
		/		
		/		
		/		
		/		
		/		

Blood Pressure Monitoring Chart

Month _____

Date	Time	Systolic / Diastolic	Pulse
		/	
		/	
		/	
		/	
		/	
		/	
		/	
		/	
		/	
		/	
		/	
		/	
		/	
		/	

Blood Pressure Monitoring Chart

Month _____

Date	Time	Systolic / Diastolic	Pulse
		/	
		/	
		/	
		/	
		/	
		/	
		/	
		/	
		/	
		/	
		/	
		/	
		/	
		/	

Blood Pressure Monitoring Chart

Month _____

Date	Time	Systolic / Diastolic	Pulse

Blood Pressure Monitoring Chart

Month _____

Date	Time	Systolic / Diastolic	Pulse
		/	
		/	
		/	
		/	
		/	
		/	
		/	
		/	
		/	
		/	
		/	
		/	
		/	
		/	

Blood Pressure Monitoring Chart

Month _____

Date	Time	Systolic / Diastolic		Pulse
			/	
			/	
			/	
			/	
			/	
			/	
			/	
			/	
			/	
			/	
			/	
			/	
			/	
			/	

Blood Pressure Monitoring Chart

Month _____

Date	Time	Systolic / Diastolic		Pulse

Blood Pressure Monitoring Chart

Month _____

Date	Time	Systolic / Diastolic	Pulse

Blood Pressure Monitoring Chart

Month _____

Date	Time	Systolic / Diastolic	Pulse
		/	
		/	
		/	
		/	
		/	
		/	
		/	
		/	
		/	
		/	
		/	
		/	
		/	
		/	

Blood Pressure Monitoring Chart

Month _____

Date	Time	Systolic / Diastolic		Pulse
			/	
			/	
			/	
			/	
			/	
			/	
			/	
			/	
			/	
			/	
			/	
			/	
			/	
			/	

Blood Pressure Monitoring Chart

Month _____

Date	Time	Systolic / Diastolic	Pulse
		/	
		/	
		/	
		/	
		/	
		/	
		/	
		/	
		/	
		/	
		/	
		/	
		/	
		/	

Blood Pressure Monitoring Chart

Month _____

Date	Time	Systolic	/	Diastolic	Pulse
			/		
			/		
			/		
			/		
			/		
			/		
			/		
			/		
			/		
			/		
			/		
			/		
			/		

Blood Pressure Monitoring Chart

Month _____

Date	Time	Systolic	/	Diastolic	Pulse
			/		
			/		
			/		
			/		
			/		
			/		
			/		
			/		
			/		
			/		
			/		
			/		
			/		
			/		

Blood Pressure Monitoring Chart

Month _____

Date	Time	Systolic / Diastolic	Pulse
		/	
		/	
		/	
		/	
		/	
		/	
		/	
		/	
		/	
		/	
		/	
		/	
		/	

Blood Pressure Monitoring Chart

Month _____

Date	Time	Systolic / Diastolic	Pulse
		/	
		/	
		/	
		/	
		/	
		/	
		/	
		/	
		/	
		/	
		/	
		/	
		/	
		/	

Blood Pressure Monitoring Chart

Month _____

Date	Time	Systolic / Diastolic	Pulse
		/	
		/	
		/	
		/	
		/	
		/	
		/	
		/	
		/	
		/	
		/	
		/	
		/	
		/	

Blood Pressure Monitoring Chart

Month _____

Date	Time	Systolic	/	Diastolic	Pulse
			/		
			/		
			/		
			/		
			/		
			/		
			/		
			/		
			/		
			/		
			/		
			/		
			/		
			/		

Blood Pressure Monitoring Chart

Month _____

Date	Time	Systolic / Diastolic		Pulse
		/		
		/		
		/		
		/		
		/		
		/		
		/		
		/		
		/		
		/		
		/		
		/		
		/		
		/		

Blood Pressure Monitoring Chart

Month _____

Date	Time	Systolic / Diastolic		Pulse

Blood Pressure Monitoring Chart

Month _____

Date	Time	Systolic / Diastolic	Pulse
		/	
		/	
		/	
		/	
		/	
		/	
		/	
		/	
		/	
		/	
		/	
		/	
		/	
		/	

Blood Pressure Monitoring Chart

Month _____

Date	Time	Systolic / Diastolic	Pulse
		/	
		/	
		/	
		/	
		/	
		/	
		/	
		/	
		/	
		/	
		/	
		/	
		/	
		/	

Blood Pressure Monitoring Chart

Month _____

Date	Time	Systolic / Diastolic		Pulse

Blood Pressure Monitoring Chart

Month _____

Date	Time	Systolic / Diastolic		Pulse

Blood Pressure Monitoring Chart

Month _____

Date	Time	Systolic / Diastolic		Pulse
			/	
			/	
			/	
			/	
			/	
			/	
			/	
			/	
			/	
			/	
			/	
			/	
			/	
			/	

Blood Pressure Monitoring Chart

Month _____

Date	Time	Systolic / Diastolic		Pulse
		/		
		/		
		/		
		/		
		/		
		/		
		/		
		/		
		/		
		/		
		/		
		/		
		/		
		/		

Blood Pressure Monitoring Chart

Month _____

Date	Time	Systolic / Diastolic	Pulse
		/	
		/	
		/	
		/	
		/	
		/	
		/	
		/	
		/	
		/	
		/	
		/	
		/	

Blood Pressure Monitoring Chart

Month _____

Date	Time	Systolic / Diastolic	Pulse
		/	
		/	
		/	
		/	
		/	
		/	
		/	
		/	
		/	
		/	
		/	
		/	
		/	
		/	

Blood Pressure Monitoring Chart

Month _____

Date	Time	Systolic / Diastolic	Pulse
		/	
		/	
		/	
		/	
		/	
		/	
		/	
		/	
		/	
		/	
		/	
		/	
		/	
		/	

Blood Pressure Monitoring Chart

Month _____

Date	Time	Systolic / Diastolic	Pulse
		/	
		/	
		/	
		/	
		/	
		/	
		/	
		/	
		/	
		/	
		/	
		/	
		/	
		/	

Blood Pressure Monitoring Chart

Month _____

Date	Time	Systolic / Diastolic		Pulse
		/		
		/		
		/		
		/		
		/		
		/		
		/		
		/		
		/		
		/		
		/		
		/		
		/		
		/		

Blood Pressure Monitoring Chart

Month _____

Date	Time	Systolic / Diastolic	Pulse
		/	
		/	
		/	
		/	
		/	
		/	
		/	
		/	
		/	
		/	
		/	
		/	
		/	
		/	

Blood Pressure Monitoring Chart

Month _____

Date	Time	Systolic / Diastolic		Pulse
			/	
			/	
			/	
			/	
			/	
			/	
			/	
			/	
			/	
			/	
			/	
			/	
			/	
			/	

Blood Pressure Monitoring Chart

Month _____

Date	Time	Systolic / Diastolic		Pulse
		/		
		/		
		/		
		/		
		/		
		/		
		/		
		/		
		/		
		/		
		/		
		/		
		/		
		/		

Blood Pressure Monitoring Chart

Month _____

Date	Time	Systolic	/	Diastolic	Pulse
			/		
			/		
			/		
			/		
			/		
			/		
			/		
			/		
			/		
			/		
			/		
			/		
			/		
			/		

Blood Pressure Monitoring Chart

Month _____

Date	Time	Systolic / Diastolic	Pulse
		/	
		/	
		/	
		/	
		/	
		/	
		/	
		/	
		/	
		/	
		/	
		/	
		/	
		/	

Blood Pressure Monitoring Chart

Month _____

Date	Time	Systolic / Diastolic		Pulse

Blood Pressure Monitoring Chart

Month _____

Date	Time	Systolic	/	Diastolic	Pulse
			/		
			/		
			/		
			/		
			/		
			/		
			/		
			/		
			/		
			/		
			/		
			/		
			/		
			/		

Blood Pressure Monitoring Chart

Month _____

Date	Time	Systolic / Diastolic	Pulse
		/	
		/	
		/	
		/	
		/	
		/	
		/	
		/	
		/	
		/	
		/	
		/	
		/	

Blood Pressure Monitoring Chart

Month _____

Date	Time	Systolic / Diastolic	Pulse
		/	
		/	
		/	
		/	
		/	
		/	
		/	
		/	
		/	
		/	
		/	
		/	
		/	
		/	

Blood Pressure Monitoring Chart

Month _____

Date	Time	Systolic / Diastolic	Pulse
		/	
		/	
		/	
		/	
		/	
		/	
		/	
		/	
		/	
		/	
		/	
		/	
		/	
		/	

Blood Pressure Monitoring Chart

Month _____

Date	Time	Systolic / Diastolic	Pulse
		/	
		/	
		/	
		/	
		/	
		/	
		/	
		/	
		/	
		/	
		/	
		/	
		/	
		/	

Blood Pressure Monitoring Chart

Month _____

Date	Time	Systolic / Diastolic		Pulse

Blood Pressure Monitoring Chart

Month _____

Date	Time	Systolic / Diastolic	Pulse
		/	
		/	
		/	
		/	
		/	
		/	
		/	
		/	
		/	
		/	
		/	
		/	
		/	
		/	

Blood Pressure Monitoring Chart

Month _____

Date	Time	Systolic / Diastolic		Pulse

Blood Pressure Monitoring Chart

Month _____

Date	Time	Systolic / Diastolic		Pulse
			/	
			/	
			/	
			/	
			/	
			/	
			/	
			/	
			/	
			/	
			/	
			/	
			/	
			/	

Blood Pressure Monitoring Chart

Month _____

Date	Time	Systolic / Diastolic		Pulse
			/	
			/	
			/	
			/	
			/	
			/	
			/	
			/	
			/	
			/	
			/	
			/	
			/	
			/	

Blood Pressure Monitoring Chart

Month _____

Date	Time	Systolic / Diastolic	Pulse
		/	
		/	
		/	
		/	
		/	
		/	
		/	
		/	
		/	
		/	
		/	
		/	
		/	
		/	

Blood Pressure Monitoring Chart

Month _____

Date	Time	Systolic	/	Diastolic	Pulse
			/		
			/		
			/		
			/		
			/		
			/		
			/		
			/		
			/		
			/		
			/		
			/		
			/		
			/		

Blood Pressure Monitoring Chart

Month _____

Date	Time	Systolic	/	Diastolic	Pulse
			/		
			/		
			/		
			/		
			/		
			/		
			/		
			/		
			/		
			/		
			/		
			/		
			/		
			/		

Blood Pressure Monitoring Chart

Month _____

Date	Time	Systolic / Diastolic		Pulse

Blood Pressure Monitoring Chart

Month _____

Date	Time	Systolic / Diastolic	Pulse
		/	
		/	
		/	
		/	
		/	
		/	
		/	
		/	
		/	
		/	
		/	
		/	
		/	
		/	

Blood Pressure Monitoring Chart

Month _____

Date	Time	Systolic	/	Diastolic	Pulse
			/		
			/		
			/		
			/		
			/		
			/		
			/		
			/		
			/		
			/		
			/		
			/		
			/		
			/		

Blood Pressure Monitoring Chart

Month _____

Date	Time	Systolic / Diastolic	Pulse
		/	
		/	
		/	
		/	
		/	
		/	
		/	
		/	
		/	
		/	
		/	
		/	
		/	
		/	

Blood Pressure Monitoring Chart

Month _____

Date	Time	Systolic / Diastolic		Pulse

Blood Pressure Monitoring Chart

Month _____

Date	Time	Systolic / Diastolic	Pulse
		/	
		/	
		/	
		/	
		/	
		/	
		/	
		/	
		/	
		/	
		/	
		/	
		/	
		/	

Blood Pressure Monitoring Chart

Month _____

Date	Time	Systolic / Diastolic	Pulse
		/	
		/	
		/	
		/	
		/	
		/	
		/	
		/	
		/	
		/	
		/	
		/	
		/	
		/	

Blood Pressure Monitoring Chart

Month _____

Date	Time	Systolic / Diastolic	Pulse
		/	
		/	
		/	
		/	
		/	
		/	
		/	
		/	
		/	
		/	
		/	
		/	
		/	
		/	

Blood Pressure Monitoring Chart

Month _____

Date	Time	Systolic / Diastolic	Pulse
		/	
		/	
		/	
		/	
		/	
		/	
		/	
		/	
		/	
		/	
		/	
		/	
		/	
		/	

Blood Pressure Monitoring Chart

Month _____

Date	Time	Systolic / Diastolic		Pulse
			/	
			/	
			/	
			/	
			/	
			/	
			/	
			/	
			/	
			/	
			/	
			/	
			/	
			/	

Blood Pressure Monitoring Chart

Month _____

Date	Time	Systolic / Diastolic	Pulse
		/	
		/	
		/	
		/	
		/	
		/	
		/	
		/	
		/	
		/	
		/	
		/	
		/	
		/	

Blood Pressure Monitoring Chart

Month _____

Date	Time	Systolic / Diastolic		Pulse

Blood Pressure Monitoring Chart

Month _____

Date	Time	Systolic / Diastolic	Pulse
		/	
		/	
		/	
		/	
		/	
		/	
		/	
		/	
		/	
		/	
		/	
		/	
		/	

Blood Pressure Monitoring Chart

Month _____

Date	Time	Systolic / Diastolic	Pulse
		/	
		/	
		/	
		/	
		/	
		/	
		/	
		/	
		/	
		/	
		/	
		/	
		/	
		/	

Blood Pressure Monitoring Chart

Month _____

Date	Time	Systolic / Diastolic		Pulse
			/	
			/	
			/	
			/	
			/	
			/	
			/	
			/	
			/	
			/	
			/	
			/	
			/	
			/	

Blood Pressure Monitoring Chart

Month _____

Date	Time	Systolic / Diastolic	Pulse
		/	
		/	
		/	
		/	
		/	
		/	
		/	
		/	
		/	
		/	
		/	
		/	
		/	
		/	

Blood Pressure Monitoring Chart

Month _____

Date	Time	Systolic / Diastolic		Pulse

Blood Pressure Monitoring Chart

Month _____

Date	Time	Systolic / Diastolic	Pulse

Blood Pressure Monitoring Chart

Month _____

Date	Time	Systolic / Diastolic	Pulse
		/	
		/	
		/	
		/	
		/	
		/	
		/	
		/	
		/	
		/	
		/	
		/	
		/	

Blood Pressure Monitoring Chart

Month _____

Date	Time	Systolic / Diastolic	Pulse
		/	
		/	
		/	
		/	
		/	
		/	
		/	
		/	
		/	
		/	
		/	
		/	
		/	
		/	

Blood Pressure Monitoring Chart

Month _____

Date	Time	Systolic / Diastolic		Pulse

Blood Pressure Monitoring Chart

Month _____

Date	Time	Systolic / Diastolic		Pulse
			/	
			/	
			/	
			/	
			/	
			/	
			/	
			/	
			/	
			/	
			/	
			/	
			/	
			/	

Blood Pressure Monitoring Chart

Month _____

Date	Time	Systolic / Diastolic		Pulse

Blood Pressure Monitoring Chart

Month _____

Date	Time	Systolic	/	Diastolic	Pulse
			/		
			/		
			/		
			/		
			/		
			/		
			/		
			/		
			/		
			/		
			/		
			/		
			/		
			/		

Blood Pressure Monitoring Chart

Month _____

Date	Time	Systolic / Diastolic	Pulse
		/	
		/	
		/	
		/	
		/	
		/	
		/	
		/	
		/	
		/	
		/	
		/	
		/	

Blood Pressure Monitoring Chart

Month _____

Date	Time	Systolic / Diastolic	Pulse
		/	
		/	
		/	
		/	
		/	
		/	
		/	
		/	
		/	
		/	
		/	
		/	
		/	
		/	

Blood Pressure Monitoring Chart

Month _____

Date	Time	Systolic / Diastolic		Pulse

Blood Pressure Monitoring Chart

Month _____

Date	Time	Systolic / Diastolic		Pulse
			/	
			/	
			/	
			/	
			/	
			/	
			/	
			/	
			/	
			/	
			/	
			/	
			/	
			/	

Blood Pressure Monitoring Chart

Month _____

Date	Time	Systolic / Diastolic		Pulse

Blood Pressure Monitoring Chart

Month _____

Date	Time	Systolic / Diastolic	Pulse
		/	
		/	
		/	
		/	
		/	
		/	
		/	
		/	
		/	
		/	
		/	
		/	
		/	
		/	

Blood Pressure Monitoring Chart

Month _____

Date	Time	Systolic / Diastolic	Pulse
		/	
		/	
		/	
		/	
		/	
		/	
		/	
		/	
		/	
		/	
		/	
		/	
		/	
		/	

Blood Pressure Monitoring Chart

Month _____

Date	Time	Systolic / Diastolic	Pulse
		/	
		/	
		/	
		/	
		/	
		/	
		/	
		/	
		/	
		/	
		/	
		/	
		/	
		/	

Blood Pressure Monitoring Chart

Month _____

Date	Time	Systolic / Diastolic	Pulse
		/	
		/	
		/	
		/	
		/	
		/	
		/	
		/	
		/	
		/	
		/	
		/	
		/	
		/	

Blood Pressure Monitoring Chart

Month _____

Date	Time	Systolic / Diastolic	Pulse
		/	
		/	
		/	
		/	
		/	
		/	
		/	
		/	
		/	
		/	
		/	
		/	
		/	
		/	

Blood Pressure Monitoring Chart

Month _____

Date	Time	Systolic / Diastolic		Pulse
			/	
			/	
			/	
			/	
			/	
			/	
			/	
			/	
			/	
			/	
			/	
			/	
			/	

Blood Pressure Monitoring Chart

Month _____

Date	Time	Systolic / Diastolic		Pulse

Blood Pressure Monitoring Chart

Month _____

Date	Time	Systolic / Diastolic	Pulse
		/	
		/	
		/	
		/	
		/	
		/	
		/	
		/	
		/	
		/	
		/	
		/	
		/	

Blood Pressure Monitoring Chart

Month _____

Date	Time	Systolic / Diastolic	Pulse
		/	
		/	
		/	
		/	
		/	
		/	
		/	
		/	
		/	
		/	
		/	
		/	
		/	
		/	

Blood Pressure Monitoring Chart

Month _____

Date	Time	Systolic / Diastolic	Pulse
		/	
		/	
		/	
		/	
		/	
		/	
		/	
		/	
		/	
		/	
		/	
		/	
		/	
		/	

Blood Pressure Monitoring Chart

Month _____

Date	Time	Systolic / Diastolic	Pulse
		/	
		/	
		/	
		/	
		/	
		/	
		/	
		/	
		/	
		/	
		/	
		/	
		/	
		/	

Blood Pressure Monitoring Chart

Month _____

Date	Time	Systolic / Diastolic		Pulse

Blood Pressure Monitoring Chart

Month _____

Date	Time	Systolic	/	Diastolic	Pulse
			/		
			/		
			/		
			/		
			/		
			/		
			/		
			/		
			/		
			/		
			/		
			/		
			/		
			/		

Blood Pressure Monitoring Chart

Month _____

Date	Time	Systolic / Diastolic	Pulse
		/	
		/	
		/	
		/	
		/	
		/	
		/	
		/	
		/	
		/	
		/	
		/	
		/	

Blood Pressure Monitoring Chart

Month _____

Date	Time	Systolic / Diastolic	Pulse
		/	
		/	
		/	
		/	
		/	
		/	
		/	
		/	
		/	
		/	
		/	
		/	
		/	
		/	

Blood Pressure Monitoring Chart

Month _____

Date	Time	Systolic / Diastolic	Pulse
		/	
		/	
		/	
		/	
		/	
		/	
		/	
		/	
		/	
		/	
		/	
		/	
		/	
		/	

Blood Pressure Monitoring Chart

Month _____

Date	Time	Systolic / Diastolic	Pulse
		/	
		/	
		/	
		/	
		/	
		/	
		/	
		/	
		/	
		/	
		/	
		/	
		/	
		/	

Blood Pressure Monitoring Chart

Month _____

Date	Time	Systolic / Diastolic		Pulse
			/	
			/	
			/	
			/	
			/	
			/	
			/	
			/	
			/	
			/	
			/	
			/	
			/	
			/	

Blood Pressure Monitoring Chart

Month _____

Date	Time	Systolic	/	Diastolic	Pulse
			/		
			/		
			/		
			/		
			/		
			/		
			/		
			/		
			/		
			/		
			/		
			/		
			/		
			/		

Blood Pressure Monitoring Chart

Month _____

Date	Time	Systolic / Diastolic		Pulse
		/		
		/		
		/		
		/		
		/		
		/		
		/		
		/		
		/		
		/		
		/		
		/		
		/		

Blood Pressure Monitoring Chart

Month _____

Date	Time	Systolic / Diastolic	Pulse
		/	
		/	
		/	
		/	
		/	
		/	
		/	
		/	
		/	
		/	
		/	
		/	
		/	
		/	

Blood Pressure Monitoring Chart

Month _____

Date	Time	Systolic / Diastolic		Pulse
			/	
			/	
			/	
			/	
			/	
			/	
			/	
			/	
			/	
			/	
			/	
			/	
			/	
			/	

Blood Pressure Monitoring Chart

Month _____

Date	Time	Systolic / Diastolic		Pulse

Blood Pressure Monitoring Chart

Month _____

Date	Time	Systolic / Diastolic		Pulse
			/	
			/	
			/	
			/	
			/	
			/	
			/	
			/	
			/	
			/	
			/	
			/	
			/	
			/	

Blood Pressure Monitoring Chart

Month _____

Date	Time	Systolic / Diastolic	Pulse
		/	
		/	
		/	
		/	
		/	
		/	
		/	
		/	
		/	
		/	
		/	
		/	
		/	
		/	

Blood Pressure Monitoring Chart

Month _____

Date	Time	Systolic / Diastolic		Pulse

Blood Pressure Monitoring Chart

Month _____

Date	Time	Systolic / Diastolic		Pulse

Blood Pressure Monitoring Chart

Month _____

Date	Time	Systolic	/	Diastolic	Pulse
			/		
			/		
			/		
			/		
			/		
			/		
			/		
			/		
			/		
			/		
			/		
			/		
			/		
			/		

Blood Pressure Monitoring Chart

Month _____

Date	Time	Systolic / Diastolic	Pulse
		/	
		/	
		/	
		/	
		/	
		/	
		/	
		/	
		/	
		/	
		/	
		/	
		/	
		/	

Blood Pressure Monitoring Chart

Month _____

Date	Time	Systolic / Diastolic	Pulse
		/	
		/	
		/	
		/	
		/	
		/	
		/	
		/	
		/	
		/	
		/	
		/	
		/	
		/	

Blood Pressure Monitoring Chart

Month _____

Date	Time	Systolic / Diastolic	Pulse
		/	
		/	
		/	
		/	
		/	
		/	
		/	
		/	
		/	
		/	
		/	
		/	
		/	
		/	

Made in the USA
Las Vegas, NV
02 December 2024

13167354R00069